YOUR KNOWLEDGE HAS VALUE

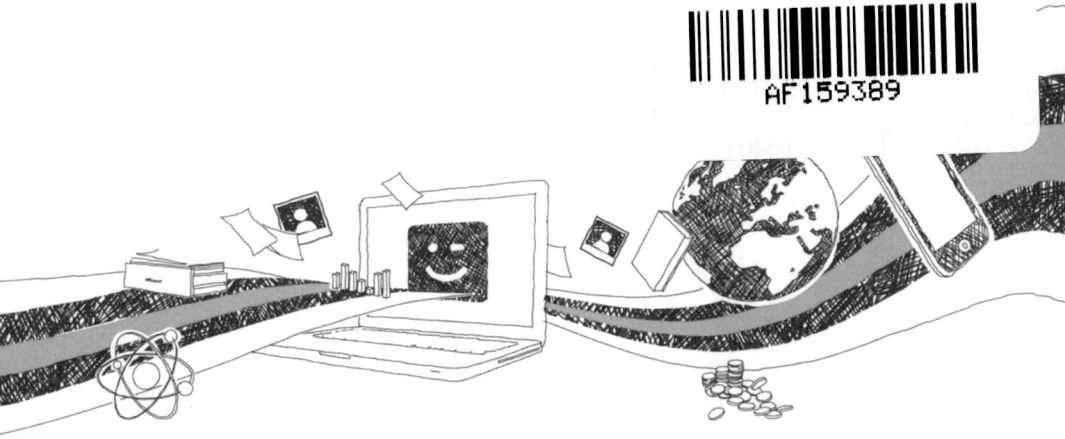

- We will publish your bachelor's and master's thesis, essays and papers

- Your own eBook and book - sold worldwide in all relevant shops

- Earn money with each sale

Upload your text at www.GRIN.com
and publish for free

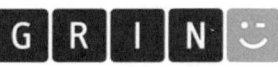

Bibliographic information published by the German National Library:

The German National Library lists this publication in the National Bibliography; detailed bibliographic data are available on the Internet at http://dnb.dnb.de .

This book is copyright material and must not be copied, reproduced, transferred, distributed, leased, licensed or publicly performed or used in any way except as specifically permitted in writing by the publishers, as allowed under the terms and conditions under which it was purchased or as strictly permitted by applicable copyright law. Any unauthorized distribution or use of this text may be a direct infringement of the author s and publisher s rights and those responsible may be liable in law accordingly.

Imprint:

Copyright © 2016 GRIN Verlag, Open Publishing GmbH
Print and binding: Books on Demand GmbH, Norderstedt Germany
ISBN: 9783668575813

This book at GRIN:

https://www.grin.com/document/381225

Patrick Kimuyu

Obesity Among Children Aged 6 to 12 Years. Causes and Risk Factors

GRIN Publishing

GRIN - Your knowledge has value

Since its foundation in 1998, GRIN has specialized in publishing academic texts by students, college teachers and other academics as e-book and printed book. The website www.grin.com is an ideal platform for presenting term papers, final papers, scientific essays, dissertations and specialist books.

Visit us on the internet:

http://www.grin.com/

http://www.facebook.com/grincom

http://www.twitter.com/grin_com

OBESITY AMONG CHILDREN AGED 6 TO 12 YEARS

Name: Patrick K. Kimuyu

Introduction 2
Epidemiology of Childhood Obesity 2
Causes and Risk Factors 2
Reason for Increased Rates of Childhood Obesity 3
Socio-economic Status Link to Childhood Obesity 3
Physical Activity and Sedentary Lifestyle 4
Neighborhood Environments and Childhood Obesity 5
Educational Status 7
Economic Status 7
Solution to Childhood Obesity 8
Conclusion 8
References 10

Introduction

Ordinarily, obesity among children aged 6-12 years is referred to as childhood or pediatric obesity and it is one of the most challenging health conditions to the global healthcare systems. Recent epidemiological studies indicate that the prevalence rates of childhood obesity have assumed upward trends in the past two decades, leading to unprecedented shorter life expectancy among the current children generation than their parents, owing to the increase of obesity related diseases burden. Research indicates that "the overall health and well-being of children is 37% lower today than it was during the mid-1970s. One of the largest contributors to children's declining health is obesity" (Sherrets & Young, n.d, p. 1).

In most cases, obese children have increased risk of growing into obese adults and this condition predisposes them to obesity related chronic conditions such as hypertension, type 2 diabetes, atherosclerosis and heart attack. Lasserre et al. (2007) state, "In children, as in adults, obesity is associated with chronic conditions such as type 2 diabetes or hypertension" (p. 157). Therefore, this research paper will provide an overview of childhood obesity, giving emphasis on socio-economic status as the principal reason why prevalence rates have increased over the past two decades.

Epidemiology of Childhood Obesity

In the past, childhood obesity was believed to be a condition among populations in the western countries, but recent epidemiological evidence shows it has crept into developing countries. It is reported, "While pediatric obesity has long been associated with western countries, accumulating evidence shows that the epidemic extends to developing countries as well, in addition to an ongoing problem of under-nutrition in the latter" (Lasserre et al., 2007, p. 157). In 2010, 35 million children in developing countries were estimated to be obese and overweight, while those who were at risk of overweight were 92 million. Globally, prevalence rates of childhood obesity had increased to 6.7% by 2010 from 4.2 in 1990. Moreover, epidemiological models indicate that the prevalence rate of obesity may reach 12.7% by 2020 (Blössner, Borghi & Onis, 2010).

Causes and Risk Factors

Research shows the principal causes of childhood obesity as the reduction of physical exercise, poor dietary habits, genetic factors and socio-economic situations. In America, where prevalence of childhood obesity, 10% 0f high school students do not engage in any physical exercise and, 65% fail to meet daily physical activity requirements; whereas 80% lack adequate fruits and vegetables in their diets (Sherrets & Young, n.d).

On the other hand, children aged 6 – 12 years have been found to have adopted a sedentary lifestyle in which they spent long hours in watching television and playing video games in computers. A survey conducted by the National Business Group on Health shows that, 25% of students use computers for recreational purposes such as playing video games for more than 3 hours daily, while 35% spent 3 or more hours watching television programs (Sherrets & Young, n.d).

Reason for Increased Rates of Childhood Obesity

Despite that, dietary habits, physical exercise and biological factors are considered as the predisposing factors for the occurrence of obesity among children, more or less the same way as in adults, all these factors have been found to be influenced by the socio-economic status of the population. A systematic review of this issue in the U.S and other countries in the European Union revealed a correlation between childhood obesity and the socio-economic status (SES) of the parents (Knott & Scott, 2015). Therefore, socio-economic status of households is the principal cause of obesity among children, especially in developed countries and urban centers in low-income countries.

Socio-economic Status Link to Childhood Obesity

The increasing prevalence trends of childhood obesity have attracted immense health concern among healthcare agencies. Charles and Lauzon (2004) reaffirm that, "Childhood obesity is a major healthcare concern, although the majority of obese or overweight children have no medical complications specific disorders can occur in the case of severe obesity and some subclinical disorders are more common in obese children" (par. 1). As a result, extensive epidemiological studies are currently on the increase to ascertain the underlying principal risk factors and, most study findings indicate that Socioeconomic Status is to blame for the unprecedented increase in childhood obesity among the global population.

It has been found out that the risk factors of childhood obesity are significantly influenced by the socioeconomic status of different households and communities and, the prevalence trends exhibit various demographic inequalities. Ordinarily, obesity is known to be among the so-called 'life-style diseases', also referred to as non-communicable diseases in clinical jargon. As such, it is highly influenced by the people's social life. In addition, economic factors have also been found to contribute significantly to the prevalence of childhood obesity, especially with regard to the income status of households in different geographical regions. Ulijaszek (2012) states, "socioeconomic status has two closely related dimensions. The economic one is represented by financial wealth while the social one can incorporate education, occupational prestige, authority and community standing" (p. 1).

It is true to assert that, the prevalence of childhood obesity among children and adolescents is influenced by the Social economic status aspect, more or less, the same way as it occurs among the adults; thus, childhood obesity and Social economic status intertwines in a synergistic manner.

Recent demographic reports indicate that, high social economic status is associated to a reduced prevalence of childhood obesity. In contrast, children from households with low social economic status have been found to be adversely affected by childhood obesity. Childhood prevalence rates are relatively high among children from communities with low social economic status, whereas those from communities with high social economic status record low prevalence rates. Ulijaszek (2012) reaffirms, "In industrialized societies, obesity is a characteristic of lower social and economic classes, having been associated with higher classes prior to widespread economic prosperity" (p. 1). This aspect is also evidenced by supported by a research report released by the Canadian Journal of Public Health, "the percentage of overweight children varied from 24% in areas with high socioeconomic status to 35% in low socioeconomic neighborhoods" (Datey, 2005, par. 4).

Physical Activity and Sedentary Lifestyle

In regard to physical inactivity among children, prevalence rates of childhood obesity are usually different between active and inactive children. Ordinarily, inactivity and sedentary lifestyle are among the predisposing factors of obesity across all ages. Charles and Lauzon (2004) explain, "the epidemic of obesity has developed concomitantly with a decrease in physical activity and an increase in sedentary activities" (par. 5). However, it is worth noting that the prevalence and incidence rates vary significantly, especially with regard to gender and professional occupations.

Therefore, prevalence trends of childhood obesity among children are immensely influence by the children's access to recreational amenities. Recent epidemiological reports reveal that access to recreational amenities influences the physical activity of children. This is evidenced by surveys, which showed that prevalence rates of obesity among children who do not have access to sidewalks are 32% likely to become obese compared to their counterparts with access to sidewalks and walking paths. In addition, access to community centers and playgrounds has been found to influence the prevalence of childhood obesity, in which the higher rates 20% and 26% respectively are reported among children with no access to these amenities compared to those who have access (Kogan, 2010).

In regard to access to health promoting amenities, prevalence rates of obesity among children with access to health promoting amenities has been found to be 20.6% compared to the increased percentage of 32.4% recorded among children with limited access to health promoting amenities. On the other hand, overweight prevalence rates have been found to exhibit the same trends, in which children with access to health promoting amenities record 38.5% whereas those with limited access to these amenities record an increased rate of 49.5% (Kogan, 2010).

However, it is worth noting that, prevalence rates of childhood obesity varies significantly between girls and boys. Girls have been found to be highly vulnerable to obesity in both situations compared to the boys. Recent health reports indicate that girls living in environments with limited access to health promoting amenities experienced an increased obesity risk of 19.2% compared to 10.4% recorded among girls with access to health promoting amenities (Kogan, 2010).

Leisure has also been found to influence the prevalence of obesity among children. Epidemiological surveys have revealed the underlying correlation between children's leisure and obesity. The time spent by children watching television programs and videos have been found to be one of the most significant determinants on the prevalence of overweight and obesity.

Children who spent the greatest percentage of their time sitting in front of televisions have increased obesity risks, compared to those who consume least time watching televisions. Kogan (2010) reaffirmed this aspect by stating, "Children who watched television more than two hours per day had 46 percent higher odds of obesity and 51 percent higher odds of overweight than those who watched television less than one hour per day" (p. 509). This occurrence has been justified with the tendency of consuming increased amounts of calories rich diets such as snacks. Moreover, the reduced percentage of time spent by these children in doing physical activities contributes to the increased incidences of obesity and overweight (Charles & Lauzon, 2004).

Neighborhood Environments and Childhood Obesity

The influence of social economic status on the prevalence of childhood obesity can be explained by the situation in the United States. Recent epidemiological reports in the U.S explain the correlation of these two elements and, the findings justify that all the risk factors for childhood obesity among the global population are related to the social economic status of different communities. However, it is worth noting that social economic status determines the social and economic aspect of the society but, the observed epidemiological disparities are attributable to an array of social and economic factors. Some of these issues include demographic changes and health transition among different communities in different regions.

In the United States, demographic factors vary significantly with regions and ethnicity; thus, prevalence trends of obesity have been studied under diverse dimensions, especially with regard to the people's neighborhood environment and social stratification of the U.S population. Neighborhood influences on the prevalence rates of obesity and overweight, in the United States, are seemingly conspicuous, especially with regard to the people's economic income and the educational level. Kogan (2010) also reports, "Neighborhood socioeconomic deprivation has also been associated with increased risks of obesity, poor diet, and physical inactivity among Canadian and U.K. children and adolescents" (p. 504). Therefore, neighborhood social economic conditions are believed to be among the principal factors enhancing the increase of childhood obesity and overweight, in the United States. Moreover, they state, "the odds of a child's being obese or overweight were 20–60 percent higher among children in neighborhoods with the most unfavorable social conditions" (p. 503). Moreover, other significant determinants of the prevalence trends childhood obesity are the 'built environments', which influence children's level of physical activity.

Epidemiological reports indicate that, childhood obesity has manifested different prevalence trends in the past decade but, there is a correlation between the risk of obesity and the neighborhood environments. For instance, in 2007, the total percentage of obese and overweight, in the United States were found to be 16.4 percent and 31.6 percent respectively, with reference to children aged between 10 to 17 years. The impact of the children's neighborhood was evidenced by the epidemiological differences in the prevalence and incidence rates of childhood obesity. In a number of epidemiological studies conducted by several health agencies revealed an unprecedented inequality in healthcare, especially with regard to the prevalence patterns of childhood obesity, in which children who were living in neighborhoods with the least favorable social conditions were found to face an increased obesity risk than their counterparts living in neighborhoods with favorable social conditions. Statistics indicated that, 37 % of children living in neighborhoods with the least favorable social conditions were overweight, whereas obesity accounted for 20% of the total population in unfavorable environments. In contrast, children living in neighborhoods with favorable social conditions recorded reduced obesity prevalence percentages, in which 29.8% were found to be overweight, whereas obese children accounted for 14.7% of the total population of children in the concerned environment (Kogan, 2010).

In general, the risk of obesity among children living in unfavorable neighborhoods was found to be 61% higher that the case recorded among children living in environments with favorable social conditions. In addition, overweight risk rates among children living in favorable neighborhoods were 43% lower compared to the increased risks in their counterparts in unsafe neighborhoods.

Educational Status

Moreover, educational status of the heads of households and the level of literacy among children and adolescents contributes significantly to the increasing trends of childhood obesity. In most cases, children from households headed by individuals less education are more likely to become obese than their counterparts from those headed by individuals with a college degree and above. This aspect is reaffirmed by epidemiological report prepared by Carroll et al. (2010) who explained, "Children and adolescents living in households where the head of household has a college degree are less likely to be obese compared with those living in households where the household head has less education" (par. 1).

Recent epidemiological studies reveal that boys and girls from households headed by an individual who education (Kogan, 2010). Therefore, it is true to state that, the prevalence of childhood obesity increases with an increase of the educational status of the head of the household possess undergraduate or graduate constitute for 11.8% and 8% respectively, whereas those from households headed by individuals with education level of undergraduate account for 21.1% and 20.4% for boys and girls respectively (Carroll et al., 2010). Further epidemiological reports show that, children from households headed by parents without a high school education were 169% likely to become obese compared to those brought up by parents who have attained college education.

Economic Status

Another social economic status aspect, which influences the prevalence of obesity among children, is the income status of different social classes in the society. Epidemiological surveys conducted by the Center for Disease Control and Prevention from

2005 to 2008 indicated that the prevalence of childhood obesity was correlated to the income status of different households and, this revelation was found to be relatively the same to the situation experienced among the adults. These surveys showed that children from low-income households recorded high prevalence rates of obesity compared to their counterparts from medium and high-income households (Carroll et al., 2010). In the CDC reports, boys from households with income status below 130% of the poverty level were found to have a higher obesity prevalence compared to those living from households whose income status were 350% of the poverty level. Statistics indicated that boys from low-income households accounted for 21.1% of the total number of obese children, by 2010, whereas those from high-income households accounted for a reduced prevalence rate of 11.9%. On the other hand, prevalence of obesity among girls living in households whose income status were below 130% of the poverty level was found to be 19.3% compared to 12.0% recorded by girls from households with incomes status above 350% of the poverty level (Carroll et. al., 2010).

In general, the total number of obese children, in the United States comprises of different percentages of children from different household categories. Children from households with income status above 350% of the poverty level constituted the lowest prevalence rate, constituting for 24% (3 million) of the total population of obese children. The remaining 78% (9 million) constituted of children from households whose income status was below 350% of the poverty level, in the U.S. However, it is worth noting that, the prevalence rates among children from households with income status categories of 350%-130% and below 130% of the poverty level were relatively the same.

Solution to Childhood Obesity

From an epidemiological perspective, there is need for designing efficient control and preventive measures to address the issue. One of the most significant preventive measures is the introduction of health programs in schools, especially with regard to the enhancement of physical activity. Secondly, educational policies should be reviewed to ensure that schools are established in healthy environments where playgrounds and other recreational facilities such as parks are accessible to children.

Conclusion

In a brief conclusion, it seems true to assert that, socio-economic status influences all childhood obesity risk factors including dietary regime and physical exercise because; the prevalence trends of the diseases correlates with the socio-demographic factors. The unprecedented increase in the prevalence of childhood obesity among the global population can be attributed to the increase of socioeconomic inequalities. Some of the most significant socio-demographic factors, which influence the prevalence of childhood obesity, are the social conditions of the so-called 'built environments', economic income status and educational status (Carroll et. al., 2010).

It is suggested that reducing the prevalence of obesity among children aged 6 to 12 years will prolong life expectancy of the current children generation. In addition, it will help to reduce the economic burden caused by obesity and its related health conditions among the global population.

References

Blössner, M., Borghi, E., & Onis, M. (2010). Global prevalence and trends of overweight and obesity among preschool children. *Am J Clin Nutr.*, *92*(5), 1257-1264.

Carroll, M., Ogden, C., Lamb, M., & Flegal, K. (2010). *Obesity and Socioeconomic Status in Children and Adolescents: United States, 2005-2008*. Retrieved from http://www.cdc.gov/nchs/data/databriefs/db51.htm

Charles, M., & Lauzon, B. (2004). Childhood Obesity: Influences of Socioeconomic Factor. *Objectif Nutrition*, 73. Retrieved from http://www.danoneinstitute.org/objective_nutrition_newsletter/on73.php

Datey, J. (2005). *Study: Socioeconomic Status and Obesity in Children*. Retrieved from http://www.statcan.gc.ca/daily-quotidien/051104/dq051104b-eng.htm

Knott, L., & Scott, O. (2015). *Obesity in Children*. Retrieved from http://www.patient.co.uk/doctor/obesity-in-children

Kogan, M. (2010). Neighborhood Socioeconomic Conditions, Built Environments, And Childhood Obesity. *Health Affairs*, 29(3), 503–512.

Lasserre, A., Chiolero, A., Paccaud, F., & Bovet, P. (2007). Worldwide trends in childhood obesity. *Swiss Med Wkly*, 137, 157–158.

Sherrets, D., & Young, J. (n.d.). *Childhood obesity: separating fact from fiction*. Retrieved from http://www.businessgrouphealth.org/pub/f312aec3-2354-d714-51ef-520ecd67dbfc

Ulijaszek, S. (2012). Socioeconomic Status, Forms of Capital and Obesity. *J Gastrointest Canc., 2012*, 1-5. DOI 10.1007/s12029-012-9366-5.

YOUR KNOWLEDGE HAS VALUE

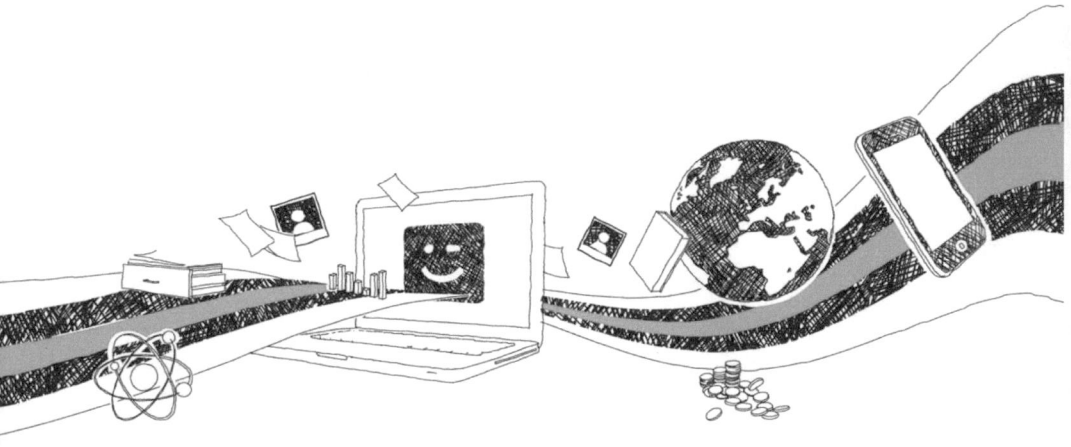

- We will publish your bachelor's and master's thesis, essays and papers

- Your own eBook and book - sold worldwide in all relevant shops

- Earn money with each sale

Upload your text at www.GRIN.com
and publish for free

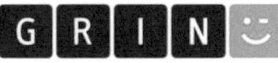